Achieving Your Healthy Weight with EFT

by
Janet Brown
Wolfbrook Holistic Healing

© 2006
Revised ©November 15, 2012
Second edition ©2017
By Janet Brown

Disclaimer: No part of this book is intended to diagnose, treat, or cure any illness. Nothing in this book is to be construed as medical advice; the author is not a doctor. Please discuss your personal health, including any options contained within this book with your personal qualified health practitioner before making any changes to your diet or medication. I and my family in perpetuity are not responsible for any adverse outcomes associated with using or misconstruing any advice or information in this book.

Most of the weight loss books out today have a few problems: they can take a long time to read, they can be boring, the methods they prescribe can be complicated and difficult to use on a daily basis.
And... they seldom consistently work.

*IF YOU TRULY WANT TO CHANGE,
THIS IS WHERE IT BEGINS:
IN THE MIND AND IN THE EMOTIONS.*

EFT (Tapping) is a fantastic tool, and used within the context of owning our personal power, the speed of our healing will be amazing, and even instantaneous.

This book will be brief as possible, to the point, and offers concrete ways to truly help. You may only want to try the EFT part, or you may want to incorporate some or all of the other health methods. At the very least, do the EFT. If you find you have problems or just can't seem to "get it", DON'T GIVE UP—you should seek the care of a professional EFT consultant.

If you do not *solve* your problem of why you keep extra weight on and have difficulty losing it, you will find it easy to regain or increase your weight; and then no weight loss plan or pill will work for you. Also, if you have problems with bulimia or anorexia, this method can work for you. If your problem is severe or chronic, please use this in conjunction with supervised medical care.

Today there are so many different types of diets, exercise programs, and self-help books it can be overwhelming to figure out which one could work for you, which one you should go with. There are many good ones out there, but few emphasize fixing the true cause behind weight loss problems and eating disorders.

How many times have you tried various forms of diets or weight loss techniques, lost a few pounds (or even maybe more!), only to gain back all or most of the weight you lost?

The reason many weight loss programs fail is because there are four things that need to be done before a person ever starts on the recommended diet or exercise plan. Find out what they are and you may succeed, no matter how many times it didn't work before.

Excess weight can be the result of many factors. In order to facilitate weight loss that is healthy and permanent, I feel a comprehensive approach is in order. So what are these four things you need to do?

The four things you need to do are:

    a. Balance the mind and emotions

    b. Cleanse the body system

    c. Build the body system

    d. Establish the life plan that is right for you

Now, most of us tend to start weight programs out of a sense of desperation (maybe even a little self-loathing) and grab the hot thing, the new thing on the market. We totally ignore the first three steps and skip straight to the fourth, but not in terms of finding the right program so much as the one that promises to take the weight off quickest, and with least effort. If you really want to lose the weight and keep it off, go through these steps in the order they are given and stay with each one until you have mastered that aspect of the process.

STEP A: BALANCE THE MIND AND EMOTIONS

This step is the most important of the four. PLEASE DO NOT SKIP THIS. It will serve as the foundation to helping you lose weight and overcome your cravings. Whenever you find yourself losing hope, having a little pain that prevents you from exercising or when you procrastinate, etc. EFT (Emotional Freedom Technique) will eliminate the negative so you can accentuate the positive. The end result will be your body *in balance*.

No matter how many gimmicks, pills, or positive affirmations we do, nothing will work with any lasting effect unless we first eliminate the negative issues we've acquired.

At the end of this book, I will present some ideas for healthier living (section D) that I personally have found to be sound and logical from my years of experience in the alternative health care field, as well as good books in the suggested reading section. But for now, we will focus on the benefits of using EFT, how to do it, and some examples and testimonials to help you better understand how to incorporate this simple procedure in your daily life

You may be surprised to know that food is one of the greatest addictive substances in the world today; sugar has been proven to be more addictive than Heroin. Addictions are usually not well treated by most professionals, people come to them for a solution, and really want to get over their dependency. However they usually go back to their earlier behavior in spite of spending a lot of time and money on the problem, which would have been eliminated if only its true cause was uncovered.

The true cause of addiction is anxiety...an uneasy feeling that is temporarily hidden, or tranquilized by some substance or behavior. Inwardly, one may have always known that the need to smoke, drink, or overeat, etc. is fueled by their need to tranquilize a level of uneasiness. But one does not directly link that feeling with the true cause of their dependency.

> --Addicts often refer to their addictions as nervous (anxious) habits
> --Addicts accelerate their use when under increased stress (anxiety).
> --Addicts will replace one addiction with another if the root cause (anxiety) is not properly addressed. For example, when one gives up cigarettes, one often then eats more, thus gaining weight.

Addictive behavior is not simply a bad habit. It is an anxiety driven need that begs for relief. The real problem is that their substance (food) or behavior (eating) only relieves the anxiety temporarily. It merely masks the problem for a while, and repeats when the anxiety reoccurs.

Another big factor in trying to lose weight is the issue of self-esteem. At least 90% of the U.S. population has a problem with low self-esteem. It's the number one thing that holds people back and prevents them from living their dreams. We often believe that we don't deserve to have the best, or to be happy. Later on, I will present a number of examples of statements to work on with EFT.

Here is an example:

Donna Gould is a diet guru's dream. She'll buy anything, try anything. In the last 35 years the Matawan New Jersey woman has starved herself, taken appetite suppressants and vinegar pills, followed liquid diets and single-food diets, had her ears stapled, sent away for patches and acupuncture gadgets, and tried most major weight-loss programs. Gould is a book publicist who has read and promoted hundreds of diet titles. Yet she still struggles with her weight, now carrying 167 pounds on her 5'3" frame. "I don't eat because I'm hungry. I eat to reduce stress, to get away from something, for instant gratification"..."It's not the diet–it's the emotional aspect of eating that has made me fail so many times.1

And EFT is one way to get to the heart of the problem, to heal the emotional wounds that produce the anxiety that cause us to overeat, to binge and purge or to starve ourselves.

Food is a basic, primitive part of our lives; it is necessary for our survival. It is only when we overeat, and eat foods that aren't good for us in order to appease our anxieties that

---

1 Better Nutrition, January 2004

we get into trouble and become overweight.

EFT gets rid of the negative emotions that can cause the anxiety and other emotions that in turn lead us to seek out food for comfort. Eradicating these excessive negative energies serves to balance the body and therefore support a healthy lifestyle. Many women, and some men, eat to not only comfort themselves emotionally, but also to change the way they look. They feel that their layer of fat is a protection against being attractive to the opposite sex.

Besides helping you to overcome anxieties that lead to overeating, EFT can help with cravings for chocolate and other foods, and improve self-esteem. Self-esteem is the most common impediment to living a successful life and has many related sub-problems of which we will soon learn. EFT is wonderful for building a strong foundation of health because of how it affects one's build up over the years of related issues and problems.

Anytime there is a physical imbalance, whether it is illness or disease or excess weight, there has first been a non-physical causative factor. Science has recently made great strides in creating the technology that can prove what healers have long known—that there is a very definite link between emotions, the mental mindset, and physical imbalance.

With weight management challenges, one has to look carefully for emotional and mental triggers for a time. We all too often end up eating NOT to have to look at what we begin to see about ourselves. If we can ever get past that point, true emotional and mental re-patterning can occur. So, for the first two weeks, pretend you are observing someone you don't know.

Just observe. Don't judge. Write your feelings down. For some people, this allows one to distance oneself from the problem. See what works for you. What you are looking for and working to observe in a detached way, are those subtle signals and triggers that PRECEDE the desire to eat all throughout the day.

Think of examples from your past. When did you begin your poor eating habits or your cravings? Was it right after a divorce? Was it when your parents divorced when you were eight years old?

Think of those things that reflect abuse, rejections, failures, fears, guilt, etc. Make a list of every past negative emotion you can think of. Include every time you had a fear, rejection, guilt, anger, shame, tears, or any other negative emotion. Include the big ones and the little ones, but keep the big ones at the top; you'll want to neutralize them first. If you can't think of everything don't worry, it isn't necessary. You can always come back to your journal later.

The next step is to use the tapping every day to eliminate these negatives. Tap three times a day or whenever a negative emotion comes up. Stop and acknowledge the emotion you are experiencing and then tap for it. Do this every day until you have reduced your negative emotions down to a two, a one, or a zero, or at the very least down to something that does not bother you anymore. Make sure you observe and note your progress every day. This will give you a sense of accomplishment and serve as a guide. Handle each emotion separately—don't lump them together.

With EFT, shifts in self-image can come much faster and much more powerfully than with conventional methods. But the changes don't happen as quickly as with phobias and some physical pains. A complete self-image change often takes weeks. It will depend on the individual, the length of time the problems have been existing, and other factors: for example, all the negativity that we've been barraged with throughout our life.

There may be stages associated with going through the process of achieving your healthy weight, similar to the stages of grief:

> **Denial** which is when you try not to think about your body, you may think, "Whatever, I may as well eat junk and be happy (or what you *think* is happy) because I'm going to die anyway."

> **Anger** comes when you see other people thinner than you are, or heavier if you are trying to gain weight. The "it's always greener on the other side of the fence" feeling. Anger may also be internally directed when you have tried many different way to

get to your healthy weight with no success. Guilt is tied in to anger.

Bargaining occurs during most diets: "Well, I'll just have *one* cookie, it can't hurt me," or "I can eat this (restricted) food because *tomorrow* I will eat better! I promise!"

Depression happens when we have tried "everything" and things feel hopeless. You may not have the money needed for special diets or operations to help you achieve your goal. You may be depressed due to bullying (adults get bullied too). If you are a woman, you may not want to lose weight because looking better could attract cat calls and unwanted attention from men. Women are also more likely to experience depression than men. Depression can also be connected to Fear, Stress, and Guilt.

Acceptance is reached when you are truly happy with your body and don't care what others think. You can ignore the commercials with super thin models and other forms of advertising that objectify women, and sometimes men. You are eating and exercising in a balanced way, with no excessive behaviors.

Not everyone experiences these stages in the exact order, or experiences all of them. These can be used as a guide to tune into your own particular feelings

and serve as a platform to begin your own
evaluation of what phrases will be best to tap on.

Remember, emotional hunger is different than physical
hunger. If you experience extreme or unusual *physical*
hunger, seek the advice of a medical professional.

The Theory, History, and Concept of EFT

The Body's Energy System

Approximately 5,000 years ago, the Chinese discovered a complex system of energy circuits that run throughout the body. These energy circuits—or meridians—are the mainstay of Eastern health practices and form the basis for modern day acupuncture, acupressure and a broad assortment of different healing approaches.

Our bodies have a profound electrical nature. Any beginning course in anatomy covers this. Shuffle your feet across a carpet and then touch an item made of metal. Sometimes you can see the static electricity that is discharged from your fingertip. This wouldn't be possible unless your body had an electrical nature to it.

If you touch a hot stove you will feel the pain instantly because it is *electrochemically transmitted* along the nerves to your brain. The pain almost instantaneously and that is why you feel pain so quickly.

In any high school chemistry class it is taught that the building blocks of ALL matter (including human bodies) are ATOMS. No one denies this fact. Nor does anyone dispute that atoms are made of ENERGY (in the form of positive and negative electrical charges)

Einstein further emphasized this point with his Theory of Relativity wherein he developed the famous formula,

Energy = Mass times the speed of light squared.

In simple terms this means that physical matter (including the human body) is MADE OF ENERGY. Thus, even though the human body may appear to be solid, its foundation is made of energy (the basis for Quantum Mechanics).

This natural fact is one of the most universally agreed upon findings in the scientific world. In general, not one scientist anywhere disagrees with it. The acceptability of Quantum Mechanics ranks right up there with the laws of gravity. However, for some unknown reason, the Western healing sciences have basically ignored it and instead have focused on the chemical nature of the body. Western medicine has not given credence to these subtle, but powerful, energy flows until recent years (as acupuncture has become more popular). Medical professionals usually don't deny that these exist, although they aren't given much notice in medical science and no weight whatsoever in psychology. They do exist and many researchers and professionals are now giving energy healing more attention.

Electrochemical messages are constantly sent throughout your body to keep it informed of what is going on. Without this energy flow you would not be able to see, hear, feel, taste or smell. Another obvious bit of evidence regarding the existence of electricity (energy) in the body are the electroencephalograph (EEG) and electrocardiograph (EKG). The EEG records the *electrical activity of the brain* and the EKG records the *electrical activity of the heart*.

These devices have been used by medical science for decades and offer further validation of the Chinese science of Energy Meridians, and the body's health based on energy flow.

Dr. Roger J. Callahan, Ph.D. is the founder and developer of the Callahan Techniques® Thought Field Therapy, and is a clinical psychologist. A graduate of the University of Michigan, he received his Ph.D. in clinical psychology from Syracuse University.

He knew about the body's amazing electrical system and the meridians. Dr. Callahan discovered, by accident, an extremely useful energy healing technique based upon these electrical principles and, specifically, acupuncture.

The following account of Dr. Callahan's first experience is a direct quote from Dr. Gary Craig:
The science behind EFT was not developed like many other discoveries. That is, it was not created in a laboratory and then tested in the real world. Instead, a stunning turn of events in the real world pointed the way first.

Here's the story. In 1980 Dr. Callahan was working with a patient, Mary, for an intense water phobia. She suffered from frequent headaches and terrifying nightmares, both of which were related to her fear of water.

To seek help, she had been going from therapist to therapist for years...with no material improvement. Dr. Callahan tried to help her by conventional means for a year and a half. He didn't make much headway either. Then one day he stepped outside the normal "boundaries" of psychotherapy. Out of curiosity, he had been studying the body's energy system and decided to tap with his fingertips under her eyes (an end point of the stomach meridian). This was prompted by her complaint of some stomach discomfort. To his astonishment, she announced immediately that her phobia was gone and she raced down to a nearby swimming pool and began throwing water in her face. No fear. No headaches. **It all went away....including the nightmares. And it has never returned.** 2

Dr. Gary Craig, who studies TFT, would develop EFT out of his knowledge of energy flow and disruptions in the human body.

EFT is really very simple: simple in concept, simple in design, and simple in procedure. However most of the time the *results* from using EFT are *simply amazing!*

The energy fields flowing through our bodies can't be seen by the naked eye, but only with high tech equipment. By analogy, you do not see the energy flowing through a TV set either. You know it is there, however, by its effects. "The sounds and pictures are your ever present evidence that the energy flow exists. In the same way, EFT gives you striking evidence that energy flows within your body because it provides the effects that let you know it is there. By tapping near the end points of your energy meridians

---

2 Callahan Techniques, 2007

*you can undergo some intense changes in your emotional
and physical well-being. These changes would not happen
if there wasn't an energy system in your body."3*

Many alternative health practitioners have found ways to
use this vital energy system to help physical healing.
Acupuncture, massage therapy, psychology, and
chiropractic are but a few of them. These methods of
healing are all beneficial and can be useful adjuncts to
healing with EFT to incorporate a holistic health way of
life.

In the next section, you will learn how to use EFT to tap
away your anxieties and balance your body's energy
system. At the very least, you will feel more relaxed and
less stressed. This works differently on each individual, as
we all come from a vast range of life experiences. If you
find that you are stumped, or this is not working for you,
don't give up! Seek a qualified EFT professional. You may
just need a different perspective, or a bit of "tweaking" on
your procedure.

---

3 EFT Manual, Dr. Gary Craig

USING EFT

The Discovery Statement
The Discovery Statement is the foundation behind EFT.
This statement says:

> *"The cause of all negative emotions is a disruption in the body's energy system."*

If we relate this to Mary's water phobia, when she was going through her fear, "the energy flowing through her stomach meridian was disrupted. That energy imbalance is what was causing her emotional intensity. Tapping under her eyes sent pulses through the meridian and fixed the disruption. It balanced it out. Once the energy meridian was balanced the emotional intensity...the ear...went away. Therein lies the most powerful thing you are ever going to learn about your unwanted emotions. They are caused by energy disruptions." 4

Keep in mind that you may want to seek out a professional EFT practitioner due to issues that you may not aware of, may not admit exist, or need to seek more advanced techniques of EFT. Please be careful when using EFT on friends or family and read again the disclaimer at the beginning of this book.

---

4 Dr. Gary Craig, Introduction to EFT

The Basic Recipe

Now we are going to analyze the discovery statement in depth. As you recall, the discovery statement says, ***"The cause of all negative emotions is a disruption in the body's energy system."***

It doesn't state that a negative emotion is produced by a wounding event that happened in the past. It is critical to notice this because most conventional psychotherapy relates past traumatic events or memories to those negative emotions. This belief is the very essence of psychotherapeutic operation. A lot of times the therapist will require the patient to relive past memories or events that are extremely painful and disturbing in order to be helped.

Fortunately, EFT does not require this method in order to be effective. It goes right to the heart of the matter, the true reason behind the negative emotion: which is the disruption in the body's energy field. As Dr. Gary Craig says, "These memories may *contribute* to an unwanted emotion...but they are not the direct *cause*. Accordingly, we don't need to spend time painfully dwelling on them."

Thus there is no substantial distress at an emotional level inherent in EFT. You will have to momentarily remember your trouble, but that is all. If any pain is encountered, a good EFT counselor will treat you immediately for that pain to reduce your stress level. This is just one instance in which EFT is a revolutionary difference from established techniques.

As a further aid to your understanding, it might help if you compare the energy flow in your body to that of a computer. As long as the electricity flows through your computer normally, everything works well. However, if you were to open up the computer and use a screwdriver to touch the connections you would definitely interrupt or redirect the electric current and an electric "zzzzzt" would take place inside. The computer would break down in some way and would display its own variation of a "negative emotion."

In the same way, when our energy systems get out of place, we experience an electrical "zzzzzt" result occurring inside of us. If we fix the electrical connection by tapping, then the negative emotion disappears.

Today's psychotherapy assumes that a person's current problems are the result of past trauma and thus dealing with the memory becomes a commonplace treatment method. However, EFT shows that there is another step involved in the healing process. This step between the memory and the emotional upset is the disruption in the body's energy system. This disruption is the exact cause of the emotional upset.

Be aware that if step 2, the intermediate step, does not take place then step 3 is *out of the question*. In other words...**if the memory does not induce a interruption in the body's**

energy system then the negative emotion can't take place. This explains why memories upset some people and not others.

With some of us, our energy systems can become unbalanced under the influence of a bad memory; other people have no such problem.

Conventional psychological treatments don't recognize the validity of dealing with the disruption of the body's energy system. This can explain why some people can actually get worse when a psychologist aims for the memory and not its cause (the energy disruption). Addressing step 1 by requiring someone to graphically relive a hurtful memory can then lead to further disruption in the internal energy field. This results in additional pain, not less. It can often make the problem worse.

When we use EFT to tap and balance the energy system, pain is eliminated and inner calm is felt, instead of the negative emotion. This induces a very quick relief since the basic cause of the problem is being handled.

"The cause of ALL negative emotions is a disruption in the body's energy system"

There are some interesting ways you can diagnose energy imbalances, however those are considered advanced methods and aren't included in this book. That doesn't mean that you still can't get results with EFT. In the next pages you will learn the Basic Recipe. It is not necessary to use all the steps given in the Basic Recipe; however one cannot know which steps will work for one person and which would work on another. Therefore it is harmless and still fast enough to perform the entire process. You will still get results. Sometimes other factors such as outside influences like environmental toxins can affect how the outcome will be. Luckily, there are ways around this, too.

Using EFT only takes a few minutes, it is painless, works rapidly and is long lasting.

The 100% overhaul concept means that you tap on ALL the endpoints set up by Dr. Craig. This concept requires that you tap near the end points of many energy meridians without knowing which of them may be interrupted. Because of this, you tap more than is needed and may tap on meridians that are flowing normally. This has no adverse effects and can't hurt to do them all. Contrarily, if you miss one or two, that won't hurt either.

If or when the Basic Recipe doesn't work, there are other fine tuning methods that can work.

It doesn't matter how long you've had the problem or how intense it is.

You don't even have to believe in EFT for it to be effective.

Before presenting the Basic Recipe, it is necessary to explain about the Setup, which deals with Psychological

Reversal (PR). PR works on self-sabotage, those nagging self-doubts in the back of your mind that say to you "no matter how good you are it won't be enough".

PR actually changes the polarity of the body's electrical system. Just like there are negative and positive terminals of a battery, the energy in your body can flow in a positive way (energy flowing A-OK) or a negative way (that zzzzt that was mentioned before, the disruption in the energy system). When you perform THE SETUP METHOD, you take care of any self-sabotage by dealing with psychological reversal and do this by changing your body's polarity from negative to positive. Now you have established a beneficial arena to enable the tapping to do its job.

EFT PROCEDURE–BASIC

DISCOVERY STATEMENT–The cause of all negative emotions is a disruption in the body's energy system.

First assess your emotional state based on a scale of 0 to 10, with 10 being the most intense and 0 being no emotional upset at all. Keeping track of your progress is critical; write down your emotion or problem along with the level of intensity.

FOUR STEPS OF THE BASIC RECIPE--

1. The Setup
2. The Sequence
3. The 9 Gamut Procedure
4. The Sequence

1. THE SETUP makes sure your energy system is properly oriented before trying to remove its disruptions. This must be corrected if the rest of the basic recipe is going to work. You repeat the affirmation 3 times while rubbing the sore spot (sore due to lymphatic congestion) (preferred) or tap the Karate Chop point (of the non-dominant hand with index and middle finger of other hand).

The affirmation: "Even though I have this ___________, I

deeply and completely accept myself"

☞It doesn't matter whether or not you believe the affirmation.

☞It is best to say it with feeling and emphasis and out loud.

If you can't find a sore spot, tap on the Karate Chop Point on the side of the hand.

2. THE SEQUENCE

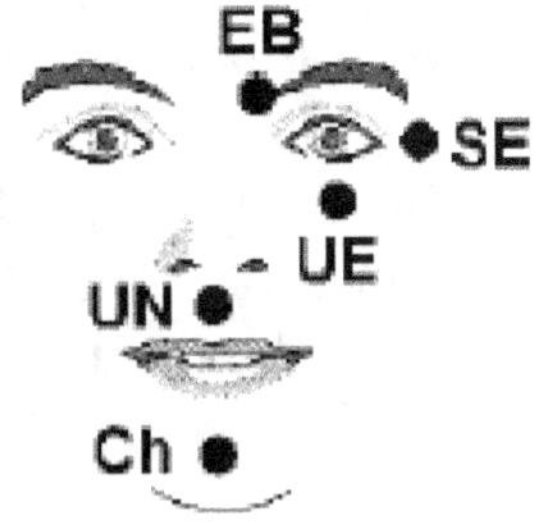

The preferred way is to tap with the dominant hand, with moderate pressure, not too lightly but do not hurt or bruise. Tap about 7 times on each point. Try not to worry if you are tapping enough times. I tell my clients that if they have a long enough phrase, like "when I got lost in the store at eight years old" by the time you've said that, you've tapped enough times. If your phrase is shorter, like "my addiction to chocolate" you keep tapping while you say the phrase twice.

It doesn't matter which side of the body you use for the tapping points. However, recent discoveries have found that if you use both hands, tapping alternately, that this can work better in most cases. If you aren't that coordinated, save that method for later. The one hand method will also work!
You are tapping on one end of the energy meridian end

points.

TH Top of Head, EB Eye Brow, SE Side of Eye, UE Under
Eye, UN Under Nose, CH Chin, CB Collar Bone
UA Under Arm (middle of bra strap for women)
L Liver point (just under the ribs, on a line down from the
breast. This will be tender)
KC Karate Chop point

These tapping points go down the body, so it is easy to
remember the sequence.

While doing the Sequence, repeat the Reminder Phrase.
Tune in to your problem. Use a word or short phrase which
describes your problem as in the affirmation. Example:
"this pain in my foot".

3. THE 9 GAMUT PROCEDURE (Do only if the above
procedure doesn't get any results)

Gamut point is between the knuckles at the base of the ring
finger and the little finger.
Do the following while tapping continuously on the Gamut
Point: Keep your head straight and
don't move it when you move your
eyes. Tune into your problem and/or
say your phrase.

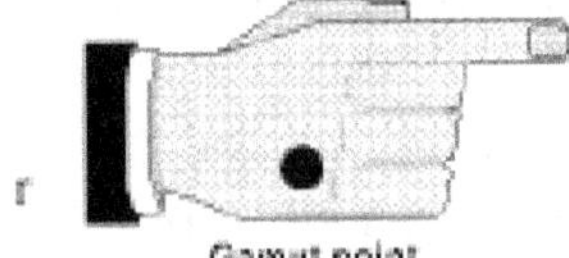

1. Eyes closed
2. Eyes open
3. Eyes hard down to the right, hold head steady
4. Eyes hard down to the left, hold head steady
5. Roll eyes in a circle, nose at center, clockwise
6. Same but now counter-clockwise
7. Hum a melody for 2 seconds
8. Count quickly from 1 to 5
9. Hum again

4. Do the "Sequence" again. Sandwich the 9 Gamut
between two Sequences.

Remember: While doing the Sequence repeat the Reminder
Phrase. Tune in to your problem. Use a word or short
phrase which describes your problem as in the affirmation.

It is important to remember these things when you are working with EFT:

> Be specific
> Be consistent
> Be personal– formulate the phrase that means the most to you

SUBSEQUENT ROUND ADJUSTMENTS

Sometimes the first time doesn't work due to a re-emergence of psychological reversal. Then you would repeat the Setup while saying:

"Even though I **still** have **some** of this _______, I deeply and completely accept myself."

Then tap while saying the reminder phrase:

"This remaining ______"

An example for all the above might be:

My craving for chocolate is at a 10.
I rub my sore spot three times, saying each time, "Even though I have this terrible craving for chocolate, I deeply and completely accept myself"
Then I tap on my endpoints, beginning with the top of the head point, and saying "this terrible craving for chocolate" at each point.

After tapping on all the points, I re-evaluate my level of
anxiety, my craving for chocolate is now at a 6. This is
good that it's gone down. However, I want this to be closer
to zero.
So I rub my sore spot again, this time saying,
"Even though I still have this terrible chocolate craving, I
deeply and completely accept myself"
Then tap saying, "This remaining chocolate craving".
My new rating is now at a 2.
I also know that if my craving level goes up, when I am
around chocolate or if I am stressed, I can tap to bring it
down.

It also helps a lot to have a piece of your favorite chocolate
to nibble on just before you evaluate to get your rating.
That way, as you lower your level down towards zero, you
can test yourself then and there with the chocolate (or other
food). You may be surprised to find how much the
chocolate loses its taste and becomes "like cardboard" as
you lower your rating.

Remember that many food addictions and weight issue
problems are attached to past abuse and self-esteem issues.
This area can be especially tricky to navigate, even more so
trying to do it yourself. If at any time you feel
uncomfortable and unsure, please CONSULT A
QUALIFIED PROFESSIONAL. EFT works fine over the
phone. The goal of EFT is not to focus on or rehash old
hurts. Sometimes these can be too painful to cope with
alone.

Jennifer5 was a forty-two year old recently divorced woman who came to me after gaining over 20 pounds due to the stress of her life with her ex-husband and the divorce that followed. Her special craving was chocolate chip cookies, especially the homemade kind, warm and fresh from the oven.

After talking with her awhile, we determined that this was definitely a "comfort craving." In her childhood, her mother had always baked and Jennifer's favorites were chocolate chip cookies and lemon bars. Her mother had passed away a few years before the divorce; Jennifer turned to her favorite comfort food to soothe the pain and stress she experienced from her mother's death and her problems with her husband.

We tapped on several issues, including the loss of her mother, her emotional abuse from ex-husband, and the stress and uncertainty surrounding the divorce. After about 90 minutes, with breaks for tissues, Jennifer had gone from a 10+ on her tapping statements down to twos and threes.

A week later she called me and was happy to report that her craving for the cookies was gone and she had begun to lose weight. Most importantly, she had regained her self-esteem and emotional strength. We had two more follow-up appointments spaced a month apart and she continued to do well. She also was excellent at using EFT on herself whenever something came up.

---

5 Names have been changed for privacy of my clients.

ASPECTS
Aspects are hidden pieces of the issue. Breaking an issue into smaller parts and Tapping on them separately is the most important key to success with EFT. These aspects are like puzzle pieces, composing the whole puzzle. Breaking a problem down into little parts and then tapping on them to their resolution is the answer to helping yourself that you may have missed.

Sometimes new aspects, related or unrelated to the problem can come up. Just apply the Basic Recipe to the new aspect until the emotional response goes to 0 (a 1 or a 2 is okay too). Don't give up. However: if you have tapped for several rounds and seem stuck on a 5 or a 4, it is perfectly ok to stop for a while. EFT will continue to work in your system, so you may find later on that your level has gone down. Also, some of us have a problem for so long and so intense that we don't recognize or know what a "0" or a "1" feels like! Just do your best! And remember, if you need help or have reached an impasse, you can always seek a professional EFT practitioner.

In order to achieve total relief on most issues, you have to confirm that EVERY Aspect has been resolved, which requires looking deeper and finding the separate parts of the issue that still needs attention.

Emotional issues can contain many different aspects. Persistence pays!

Usually the more aspects an issue has, the longer it may

take to solve them with EFT. Many times, after addressing and resolving one Aspect, your system will automatically shift to the next Aspect that needs to be addressed.

Remember to be as specific as possible. Playing a "mental movie" of the event related to your statement can help tune into the problem.

It's ok to have your eyes open for a regular course of tapping, but some prefer to close theirs. Do what feels right for yourself. Sometimes looking in the mirror helps because you can look right into your eyes, which increases the impact tapping can have and makes your statements more meaningful.

Now that you've gotten the concept for the Discovery Statement and practiced the Basic Recipe, keep practicing. And once again, if you just can't seem to get your comfort level down to a 1 or a zero (on a scale of 0 to 10), then you may need to seek the care of an EFT certified professional consultant. She or he will be able to pinpoint the problem and focus on the correct type of EFT technique, or use some advanced techniques. They will also be able to guide you in using these methods to better help yourself. That being said, a good EFT practitioner will "get themselves out of the way": they should not insist on using their own statements (other than as examples), or any incidents or emotions other than *what is personal to you!*

Sometimes all you have to do is change what you say for your Setup statement. One woman who came to see me tried, over and over again tapping on her addiction to Coke (the soft drink, not the other drug), but to no avail. She might stay off of it for up to two weeks, but then she would get the desire to have one and then go back to drinking them every day. She knew that they were ruining her health and lowering her immune system, but that was not enough reason to stop.

Her statements would be "even though I have this craving (addiction) to sugar..." And "even though I have this addiction to Coke..." For some reason, they just weren't working.

Then, in her last session, she finally hit upon the key. While thinking about her setup statement, she thought back to her childhood. Every day after coming home from school, she would have a coke and potato chips for a snack. When she tuned into this scene, tears came (when tears come, you know you've hit on something!). It was possibly the comfort associated with eating and drinking those particular items, or possible an untouched emotion wrapped around a certain event, or what a parent had said–these remained in her subconscious.

The end result for this round of tapping was that the cravings for Coca Cola were gone completely. She hasn't had even a sip of Coke for over a month. And, the truest test of all, she can even think of a Coke, and try to recreate the taste sensations of what she would experience when she really, really wanted one (how cold it was, the snappy sharpness of the bubbles, the sweetness) but not a hint of desire for one is present. This is an example of what a breakthrough treatment EFT can be–for addictions, cravings, fears–just about anything.

Here are some suggestions of setup statements to use in the area of weight loss. Remember, find what is most relevant to you and then it will work the most effectively. Also remember that food is often tied to emotions and emotional events in our childhood that can act as a trigger for weight gain. This [Setup] statement is not some form of 'magic incantation' and there is no perfect form of it for each specific problem that always works for that problem. Rather the 'Setup' statement is personal and specific to the individual sufferer. So feel free to re word the pertinent statement(s) to fit your feelings or situation.

While there are some occasions where the Set-up statement should be very specific, the only guideline necessary is that the *Setup statement must be a phrase that adequately tunes you into the problem*. Thus, the Setup statement is a simple art and does not reduce down to a library of exact phrases.

To point up an extreme example, it is no use at all to have a four year old child recite the 'Set Up' – "Even though I suffer from enuresis, I fully accept and love myself". Instead the statement must be in their own words. In this case a statement such as "Even though I wet the bed, Mummy loves me" would be a lot more effective as the child would understand what he or she was saying. For an

older child with the same problem a 'Set Up' statement
such as "Even though I'm not dry at night, I am still a cool
dude" may fit the bill. The actual form of words is not
important as long as the person's subconscious understands
what is intended.

SUGGESTIONS:
***Take note of all the statements that apply to you.

***Keep a diary of what statements you used on each day
and how you felt, your success, etc.

***Please don't tap on more than 4 or 5 different aspects at
the same time. It gets too confusing. When one issue
reduces down to below a "2" rating, or you don't have a
strong emotional reaction anymore, craving is gone, etc.,
then you can stop tapping on that particular area.

***Remember to always end your statement something
like: "I deeply and completely love and accept myself" or "I
like myself". There will be more information later on what
to do if you feel you don't like or love yourself, or can't
even say "accept".

Here are some examples of statements to tap on, divided by category. There will be a few that have no set category, I have placed them at the end; and a few will cross over and have multiple themes. If you are too thin and want to gain weight, use these statements as a "jumping off point" to inspire your own statements.

1. SUGAR AND CHOCOLATE
"Even though I crave this chocolate, I deeply and completely accept myself."

"Even though I have these chocolate cravings…"

"Even though I can't resist the Godiva chocolate, I deeply…

"Even though I crave eating sweets, especially when I'm anxious…I deeply and completely accept myself anyway."

"Even though I reach for sweets because I think they'll make me feel better…"

"Even though eating sweets feels like a reward, I deeply…"

"Even though I crave sweets in the afternoon, I deeply and completely accept myself anyway."

"Even though I always want M&M's (or whatever your favorite candy/food is) every afternoon, I deeply and

completely..."

2. DEPRIVATION

"Even though I feel deeply deprived, I completely love and accept myself."

"Even though I feel deprived because of the pressure at work..."

"Even though I overeat when I feel deprived..."

"Even though we don't have enough quality time together..."

"Even though I don't want to give up my favorite food..."

"Even though I will miss the taste of my favorite food..."

"Even though I'll feel deprived if I give up my chocolate..."

"Even though I'm afraid I won't feel safe without my food..."

"Even though I fear feeling deprived, and don't want to give anything up ..."

"Even though I feel grief when I think of losing weight,

and giving up my favorite foods...."

"Even though I don't feel safe without the extra pounds..."

3. SELF ESTEEM

"Even though I don't feel comfortable losing the weight again..."

"Even though it's a fact I'll end up wrinkled..."

"Even though I felt ashamed of my body and the extra weight..."

"Even though I'm convinced I can't lose weight and look good...

"Even though I'm never successful at what I want to do...and the more I want it the less able I am to accomplish it..."

"Even though I don't feel safe when I'm successful...I'm afraid to lose more weight..."

"Even though I feel the pressure to be perfect...."

"Even though I'm not perfect but want to be..."

"Even though I wish I could accept myself as not perfect..."

Use while tapping down the face: "I choose to accept
myself even though I'm not perfect"

"Even though I hate fat people because they're not
perfect...and NEITHER AM I..."

"Even though I hate fat people because they resent me
and disapprove of me..."

"Even though that image disgusts me, I deeply…."

"Even though it's the truth that I'll look old and
wrinkly if I lose weight…"

"Even though I'm tired of having to prove myself in
front of my boss..."

"Even though I miss my husband's attention..."

"Even though I feel inadequate, and my body's not
enough..."

"Even though I hate my body..."

"Even though I'm mad at him/her for shaming me...."
and

"Even though I forgive him/her for shaming me..."

"Even though I feel fat, and always have, I deeply love

and accept myself anyway."

"Even though I believe I'm fat...Even though I'm convinced I'm too big..."

"Even though I feel huge and fat now when I look at myself..."

"Even though I hate my body, and don't accept my body, I deeply and completely accept myself ANYWAY."

"I deeply and completely accept myself even if I never get over this problem/ never lose the weight."

"Even though I'm afraid to change..."

"Even though I'm afraid to step into my power... (I can feel safe stepping into my power)"

"Even though I've never been good enough because I'm not perfect...I AM good enough"

"Even though I let myself get distracted so I can avoid my power..."

"Even though I think I'm a fraud so I block my power..."

"Even though I'll never be enough, there was never enough, and there probably won't be enough...I choose to feel satisfied anyway.”

4. MOTIVATION

“Even though I can’t picture myself reaching my goal.”

“Even though I don’t feel safe leaving my comfort zone…”

“Even though I feel more comfortable staying overweight…”

“Even though I’m having difficulty seeing myself at my goal weight, I deeply and completely…”

“Even though I’m still having some difficulty seeing myself successfully reaching my goal weight…”

“Even though I don’t feel safe leaving my comfort zone of weight…”

“Even though I’m afraid to leave my comfort zone...”

“Even though I have this fear of leaving my comfort zone…”

“Even though I feel more comfortable staying where I am...”

“Even though this weight loss stuff is going too slow…,”

"Even though I seem to be at a plateau..."

"Even though I can't eat like others..."

"Even though I need to exercise more than twice a week..."

"Even though my body doesn't want to let go/ wants to hold on to the weight..." and "Even though my body refuses to leave this plateau..."

"Even though I dread exercising..." or "Even though I resist exercising more than twice a week..."

"Even though I'm frustrated and mad at myself that I've got to go through this again...I deeply and completely love and accept myself anyway."

"Even though I'll probably gain the weight back like I always have..."

"Even though (no matter what) it has to be a struggle to keep the weight off..."

"Even though I believe I always have to be on guard or else I'll gain it back..."

"Even though I have terrible cravings..."

"Even though I have this terrible craving to eat my favorite food, I deeply and completely accept myself"

"Even though I can't resist _______, I deeply..."

5. FAMILY

"Even though I'm afraid to look like my grandmother...

"Even though I'm afraid to be anything like my grandmother

"I forgive my grandmother for being so mean and critical..."

"Even though my father hated how and what I ate..."

"Even though my father criticized me for being overweight as a child..."

"Even though my father wanted me to exercise instead of reading books..."

"Even though I wasn't accepted for who I am..."

"Even though he never accepted me for who I was/am..."

"Even though I can't be successful without my mother's support..."

"Even though she won't give me her support if I'm

successful..."

6. GUILT Where do we learn Guilt? Most of the time, it's from our family upbringing. Scolding, shame, punishment (both mental and physical) are and have been an unfortunate part of childhood. Guilt always seeks punishment of one form or another. Anger and fear are root causes of guilt and could be aspects to tap on. Once we learn that, as adults, we continue the punishment our parents gave us whenever we feel guilty or we did something wrong, we can begin to overcome past traumas and heal.

"Even though I know I'll feel guilty if I lose more weight and my mother stays fat..." (FAMILY)

"Even though I feel guilty now because I lost weight and she feels uncomfortable..."

"Even though I still feel guilty about being thinner than my mother..." (See also FAMILY)

"Even though I feel guilty EVERY time I eat..."

"Even though I feel guilty spending money on food...I deeply and completely accept myself anyway."

"Even though I'm ashamed of myself...and my body...and for being overweight...I deeply and completely accept myself anyway."

"Even though I want to release the guilt about overeating..."

7. BREADS

"Even though I crave carbohydrates...,"

"Even though I overeat in front of the television, I deeply and completely accept myself."

8. STRESS

"Even though I eat when I feel overwhelmed by stress, I deeply love and accept myself."

"Even though I need to eat to relax and feel calm, I deeply..."

"Even though stuffing myself calms me down, I deeply..."

"Even though overeating feels soothing after a long hard day..."

"Even though I can't feel relaxed unless I'm eating/overeating..."

"Even though I give food too much power and I'm tired

of being anxious all the time...”

“Even though I don’t feel safe letting down my guard...”

“Even though I still feel unsafe about getting thinner...”

“Even though THEY won’t feel safe if I lose more weight...”

WHEW! I bet you didn’t realize there were so many emotions surrounding the topic of weight! And there are more than the ones listed above.

At this time, take a few minutes to think of your own statements to tap on. List them separately on a piece of paper; keep a journal of your tapping statements. If things get too overwhelming, emotional, or powerful please stop. Take a deep breath and go for a walk if you can. If anything is too intense to handle on your own please make an appointment with a qualified EFT counselor.

THE FORGIVENESS SET UP

Forgiving yourself (for allowing things to happen to you) is another way to heal from body image issues. The forgiveness set up simply adds the word "forgive" to an appropriate statement while you rub your sore spot.

Some examples are:

> "I forgive myself for being overweight"
> "I forgive myself for being ashamed of myself"
> "I forgive myself because I feel this is all my fault"etc.

You can change your set up statement slightly to include the word "forgive". "Choosing" is another extremely useful word to add, as in:
"Even though I eat too much, I now choose to eat less"

If you can think back to what happened the last time you were at your goal or ideal weight, this can help you identify the source of your emotional resistance to picturing yourself successfully reaching your ideal weight. Or, if you were never at an ideal weight, try to visualize yourself at that weight and imagine what others might say or do. And imagine your feelings or reactions to this.

How are you sabotaging yourself? Sometimes, women fear the extra attention from men if they were to be more slender, more "attractive". This fear alone is a very common one. Some women will associate their ideal weight with an unpleasant marriage, or possibly when their Mother or Aunt was always nagging them to be thin.

"I forgive myself for being overweight..."
"I now choose to release the pain from my childhood (or past)"

Think to yourself, "with this weight that I am at now, I know who I am, I am comfortable...what would I really be like if I changed and lost the weight?" This is an important fear that is uncovered.

("I forgive myself for being overweight...for being ashamed of myself...") while rubbing the sore spot or tapping on the Karate Chop Point.

You can use the forgiveness statement with other aspects of weight, "I forgive myself for not eating..." "I forgive myself for eating too little..."
Sometimes we associate events in our life with weight issues. *And sometimes these events are painful.*
Therefore, we associate pain with being at our ideal weight.

Another effect is carrying over punishment from our childhood. If you were punished a lot and your childhood punishments were related to or associated with food, self-esteem and body image, then as an adult, we can't live without that punishment.

So what happens? *We punish ourselves.*

We punish ourselves in ways based on those traumatic events from childhood: and most revolve around food and body image, which produces a lack of self-esteem. Sometimes we associate events in our life with weight issues and sometimes these events are painful. Therefore, we associate pain with being at our ideal weight.

> *When I was seeing Hailey as a client, she was coming from a place of emotional abuse in her childhood. She would get bullied at school as a child due to her being overweight. But this is not her fault, her mother, who had grown up during the Great Depression, made her clean her plate at every meal. Being too full made Hailey lethargic and she would retreat to her room where she could read and escape into fantasy worlds.*
>
> *Through using EFT, she began to realize where the causes were for her long-standing and deep-seated problems with food. We tapped on her relationship with her mother, the control issues she had and how her mother's beliefs of scarcity she acquired during the Depression led her to be fearful and impart those fears onto her children. We also tapped on her about her father, who fully supported her mother, and her brother, who was one of the first children to tease her about her weight.*
>
> *With a few more sessions of tapping on her self-esteem issues and some guidelines for exercise and healthy eating, Hailey enjoyed an impressive weight loss. Her enthusiasm for her new self allowed her to*

keep off the weight that had plagued her and enable her to continue, years later, to be successful in her keeping off the pounds.

A purely emotional eater uses food to numb out feelings of anxiety, stress, loneliness, grief, etc. Also overeating when in a joyful or celebrating mood:

I ate to stuff any emotion I didn't want to feel.

I feel that there are three main emotional reasons for weight issues: Self Punishment, Protection, and Self Esteem. And while these have been mentioned previously in this book, it is so important that it bears repeating!

✧**Self-Punishment** occurs especially in the areas of Bulimia and Anorexia. This includes *Deprivation,* and *Abuse or Punishment.* If, as a child, you were abused or abnormally or unusually punished this can so injure the psyche that, as an adult now living on your own, you still continue that abuse and punishment *to yourself* because your parent(s) are no longer there to do it to you. Your self worth has been so torn down that you feel that "being normal" involves some level of abuse. We punish ourselves in ways based on those traumatic events from childhood and most of those revolve around food and body image, which produces a lack of self-esteem.

✧**Protection** means feeling safe. For some of us, we cope with past abuse by protecting that child. How we protect

ourselves comes in many different forms. Some people retreat into a fantasy world. Others split off into different personalities. Some use food for protection and a sense of self-worth. Every time there is an emotional upset, food is used to comfort and placate our souls.
Another aspect of protection by overeating can be seen as making ourselves too "ugly" or unattractive so that the abuser will leave us alone.

✧**Esteem.** Esteem is definitely intertwined with the above coping mechanisms. Anything negative that we were told as a child sticks with us. It gets "written on our walls". Over time, all that negativity builds up to create the house we live in. Is your house full of negativity or full of joy? Even what seems like a harmless offhand remark can have a lasting negative impact–on a child or an adult.
EFT helps erase those negative writings, so we can then replace them with positive ones, and build a house of joy.

Your self-esteem is what you think others think of you.

Sometimes, you keep gaining weight to be "enough":
 ...Enough of a person
 ...Good enough
 ...Successful enough
 ...Pretty enough
 ...Talented enough, etc.
But at the same time, you tell yourself, "I'm never going to be good enough" or "I'll never be good enough for my (Mother/Father/Husband/Boyfriend/Teacher/Priest/Friends, etc.) So you keep gaining weight to be enough.

All or some of the above main areas combine to affect us with negative eating habits, whether they are bulimia, overeating, or anorexia.

Deprivation can be an important area for weight loss.

You might be undermining your personal weight loss to protect yourself from success and felt trapped by certain limiting beliefs about your success.

Sometimes we tell ourselves, ***"if only I could lose this weight...then I could be successful."***

"If I lose the weight, I'll have to excel at what I want to do." This puts pressure on us and makes us want to stay in our comfort zone.

FEAR is a common element of failure. We fear what we don't know and this makes us also want to stay comfortable, even if the comfort zone is not ideal for us!

We are often uncomfortable to reach out and go where we fear. We fear success and a lack of control. We want to be safe, therefore we create our own "comfort zone" whereby we cushion ourselves from the fear of the unknown, or the imagined known, the "what ifs" that always hold us back. We think that things will be difficult to handle when we lose weight, so therefore we retreat from it rather than dealing with it. EFT can help you cut out the negative patterns and then help you establish positive new patterns such as:

1. "I feel in control of myself and my eating."
2. "I no longer feel fearful of food."
3. "I don't have any more guilt after I eat."
4. "There's no more body hatred or severe
   self-criticism."
5. "I am enjoying food more than ever."

✶Stop and acknowledge the emotion you are experiencing
and then tap for it.

✶Once EFT eliminates the negative emotions, you can then
incorporate positive affirmations into your life–and they
will work 100 times better than they would have before.

You can tap the positive affirmations in to your system the
way you tapped away the negativity.
Instead of saying, "Even though..."

Say: "I now choose to eat healthy foods..."
"I now choose to love and accept my body..."
"I forgive myself for making poor food choices in
the past"
"I am healthy and happy and strong"   etc.

And I love the following, from Louise Hay:
"I go within to effect the cure. I go within to
dissolve the pattern that created this and I accept healing in
any form"
"It is easy for me to reprogram the computer of my

mind. All life is change and my mind is ever new. I am the loving operator of my mind."

WHAT TO DO IF YOU CAN'T SAY "LOVE"

In the setup statement are the words "I deeply and completely love and accept myself". Well, what do you do if you choke on these words, if you feel you are not good enough and can't "love" or even "like" and "accept" yourself?

Here are some thoughts and tips on this:

Before you do anything else, use these Setup Statements:

"Even though I have trouble loving or liking myself, I am going to try doing so now"

"Even though I feel I don't deserve to be loved, I now choose to try to like myself"

"Even though I don't like myself, I know sometimes I can be a good person"

"Even though I can't bring myself to even say "I love myself", I am going to try my best and see what happens"

These are just a few suggestions. Play around and come up with your own. Use words like "try" "I choose to" and "comfortable". Find words which will be helpful for you but not make you "close up" or "turn off." Be aware that the aspect of low self-esteem can carry tons of emotional baggage that you may not be ready to deal with. If you experience too much emotional pain, please seek the help of a professional.

TAPPING THROUGHOUT YOUR LIFE

What is *tapping throughout your life*?

Well, this means that you tap on all aspects of your problem as it specifically relates to TIME. Tap on your Present, your Past, and your Future. This is a convenient way to organize your tapping plan. Present tapping can lead the way to revealing Past issues to tap on; Future tapping can help you maintain your goals and give you a feeling of confidence.

The Present: Tap on phrases currently related to your weight. These would involve your cravings, your binging, your obsessions, and what you like as comfort foods. Be specific and refer to the examples given previously.

For example:

"Even though I crave chocolate as a snack…" (Addiction)
"Even though I hide my snacks from my family…" (Guilt)
"Even though I hate myself for eating so much…" (Self-hatred)

The Past: This area will involve as many of your past incidents of low self-esteem, family battles centering on food, your sense of self-worth as seen through the eyes of others and what derogatory things they have said to you. When do we lose our sense of self-esteem? Why is it so fragile? Why do we let others dictate to us how we feel? You can refer to the examples given previously, or use

these:
"Even though I feel unsafe without food…"
"Even though my parents scolded me at dinnertime…"
"Even though my father abused me at dinner…"
"Even though I need to eat to feel better about myself…"
"Even though I'm ashamed of my ______________" fill in the
blank with whatever body part(s) you are ashamed of.

The Future
How would you feel tomorrow or next week if you knew
today that you wouldn't be binging on food, or eating
several candy bars a day? Ask yourself this question, or one
similar to it, and note your response. Do you feel irritated?
Anxious? Lonely? Depressed? Whatever you feel, tap on
that emotion until it becomes lower than a "4".

For example:
Picture yourself being at your ideal weight. What do you
feel?
"Even though I don't deserve to be so thin…"
"Even though guys will stare at me because I'm so thin…"
"Even though people will be jealous of me because I look
so good…"

These things take time, in some cases. Don't get frustrated
if you don't get immediate results. Just keep trying and
hang in there! You can do it!

Sometimes you may not be able to pinpoint the exact
reason for your overeating, or your craving for sweets or
carbs. In that case, it's perfectly ok to begin with something

general:

"Even though I have this block to losing weight…"

"Even though I don't know why I can't lose these last 20 pounds…"

There are so many different things one could say to help with weight issues, it all depends on your particular situation. The general categories of problems that occur with everyone are:

Self-esteem, shame, guilt, and anxiety.

Find your key, specific phrases and you will be well on your way to health and healing!

RAISING THE BODY'S METABOLISM WITH EFT

EFT is a good way to raise the body's metabolism rate in order to burn more calories, whether at rest or exercising, or going about daily activities. As long as you follow the instructions carefully, and don't try to raise your metabolism too much at once, you should experience a safe and definite increase in your energy level and calorie burning level.

If you have trouble doing or saying any of the following, please seek the help of a professional EFT consultant.

It can be difficult to rate your initial metabolic rate, but similar to the SUDS rating for other EFT work, you should rate your metabolism at a percentage, such as 25%, if feeling very tired, having to take a nap during the day, etc.

The following technique can be used in the morning as a quick pick me up and boost to the day ahead. It can also be done at any time that you need more energy.

IMPORTANT—do not raise your metabolism any further than is safe for you at this time. State clearly that you are looking for your own personal 100% and you can stay within the safe limits. Don't turn it up any further than is desirable, given the conditions of the rest of your systems at this time.

As you would with working out, you build your metabolic rate gradually step by step over a period of time so that you can get used to it easily and properly.

1. Choose what level in percent your body is functioning at. Just guess or let a number come to you. Trust your intuition. There is no need to be 100% accurate, this just gives you a comparison number for later.

2. FIRST ROUND OF TAPPING–"Even though my body runs at only XX percent, I deeply and completely love and accept my body"

3. SECOND ROUND–"I want to release everything that slows my body down and I deeply and completely love and accept my body."

4. THIRD ROUND–"I want to repair everything that slows my body down and I deeply and completely love and accept myself."

SUBSEQUENT TAPPING–There may be some other things or issues that have come up since the first day of tapping. These might be memories related to your body, problems with food or diet and any thoughts or behavior. Now you can use Astra Johnston's Gauge work*:

1. Imagine a 100% gauge, similar to the speedometer on your car, which represents the *perfect* level of functioning for your own unique metabolism this moment.

2. Take a reading of how your metabolism feels right now.

3. Treat the gauge with an opening statement of your

choice, such as "I want my metabolism to function perfectly and deeply..."

4. Repeat until you have either reached the 100% or you feel that you are happy and want to stop.

Regular use of this protocol will boost your energy levels and give you a whole new sense of self-esteem all over. You can use your increased energy to further your health, your goals, your work, creativity, relationships, etc.

This is it for the first time. Take a SUDS reading, write it in your workbook, and then see how you are feeling over the next few days.

ABOUT SLEEPING

Often what happens when people boost their metabolism in this way is that they find they can't go to sleep at night; they are too energetic.

You now need less sleep because you are stronger, less exhausted and your body is running more efficiently. If this is too unnerving for you or if you think this is a problem, you can fix this in a simple way.

All you have to do is to use EFT to calm yourself in the same way as you revved up your metabolic rate in the first place. Just tap for calm, relaxation, restfulness.

Those with high metabolic rates can sleep very soundly and still keep their higher metabolic functioning in place. Most of us end up in bed at the end of the day overly exhausted and sometimes "too tired to sleep". Now, with your metabolism operating properly and optimally, you can sleep simply because it's the right thing to do.

Please keep in mind that all the stimulating things you used to do (caffeine, entertainment, food) to get you through the day will now be added into your higher metabolic rate, possibly resulting in overstimulation. You may have to reevaluate your lifestyle and make some adjustments to avoid this.

Raising your metabolic rate makes you faster, stronger and

more efficient in mind and body. EFT achieves this by taking out blockages and reversals that are slowing down the metabolism and is therefore safe and ecological.

If you get ill, simply replace the word "metabolism" with "immunity" or "my immune system." This should help your immune system fight off the cold or flu.

STICKING TO YOUR WEIGHT LOSS PLAN

Here are some tapping suggestions for staying on your eating and exercise plans. Remember, these are only suggestions!

"Even though I feel like eating junk food right now..."

"Even though I don't feel like walking (hiking, or jogging, or swimming, or biking, etc.)...."

"Even though I'd rather lie around and be lazy..."

Now, try to come up with a few of your own procrastinating statements:

Taking care of the things that are causing your health to be less than optimal should come before you start actively trying to lose weight. Give your body the emotional support it needs to lose weight, or gain weight, and you will not fail. That is why EFT is so important. It can eliminate the negative emotions behind eating problems and it can help you control cravings. EFT can help you boost your metabolism so you are more energetic and burn more calories. It can also get rid of negative eating habits such as

       "Even though I always seem to want junk food..."
Or   "Even though I can't get into juicing, it seems so difficult and involved..."

Try it on every aspect of your self-improvement and see

where it takes you! Remember to also tap on the positive aspects after eliminating the negative ones.

WHAT TO DO IF THE BASIC RECIPE DOES NOT WORK

1. Energy toxins could be the culprit. This is something to try only if the Basic Recipe isn't working for you at all.

Energy toxins aren't always things that are generally known to be bad for you. Believe it or not, what seems like healthy food can sometimes be interfering and troublesome to your energy system. One person, for example, could have citrus fruits toxic to their body's energy system.

Things you consume a lot of will tend to be energy toxins for you, even if they are healthy (peas, fruit, carrots, meat, etc.)

Other things that can be toxic to your energy system include: perfumes, dyes, herbs, wheat, corn, coffee, tea, refined sugar, dairy, alcohol, nicotine, pepper.
Eliminate these for a week and then see if the Basic Recipe works for you. If that doesn't work and you've been faithful about eliminating all the common toxins, then ask your intuition what could be interfering.

2. You give up too early, or don't keep tapping.
Not everyone wants to "do their homework" and tap on themselves outside of the therapist's office. Some people try tapping on themselves but do not experience the same progress that they do if someone else (therapist taps on them).
When this occurs, it is important to return to your EFT

practitioner for further sessions. If you want to keep tapping on yourself, then remember the cardinal "rules":

> Be specific
> Be consistent
> Be personal– formulate the phrase that
> means the most to you

Remember to tap on the different aspects or "offshoots" of the main topic.

Everyone hides things from themselves; they don't want to admit certain things. That is why tapping on oneself can be problematic. There can be a real maze of related situations that a good EFT therapist will be able to allow you to see, guide you through, and resolve.

Finding the core issues

You can begin by tapping on your immediate symptoms, cravings and feelings, and that will help. But what you also need to do is to be a detective and search out what the hidden meanings and causes could be behind your eating habits. If you need to gain weight, what could the underlying causes be in your life or in your past?
If you need to stick to an exercise plan, what is your deep-seated reason for procrastination?

Many of our core issues are rooted in past events, and many of these are entrenched in our past family dynamics. When we were children, we didn't know how to behave, we learned things from how our parents behaved. If one or both parents did not get the coping skills from their parents, or it they experienced abuse when they were children, the trickle down effect may result in problems in your current life.

No one is perfect, nor should they be. But using EFT can guide us to a better understanding of our past, and help us realize why we are the way we are. And EFT can even help us forgive the past and those that hurt us if we are ready to do so.

NUTRITIONAL METHODS TO HELP YOU

Step B.   CLEANSE THE BODY SYSTEM

The following should be taken into consideration of how
you are feeling, your doctor's opinion and your own on
your health, your eating habits, etc.

Everyone is different in body structure, metabolism, genetic
disposition, and the desire to take things to the next level;
your will power and determination.
Also, you do not necessarily need to do ALL of these in
order to be healthy. They are presented here for your
information only. New techniques and supplements are
discovered every day in the area of alternative health care.
Keep up to date by consulting books, magazines and
reliable websites on the internet. Resources are listed at the
end of this book.
When you ask the body to release something (like extra
weight) you need to give it all the support to do so.
cleansing the various systems of the body frees up more
energy for weight management.

1. **Colon**. If you are not having two to three good bowel
movements every day, you most likely have a toxic colon.
If the colon is not fully expelling the waste that gathers
there after each meal, that waste turns rotten and toxic. The
toxic waste leaks back through the wall of the colon and
back into the bloodstream. This produces a universally
unhealthy condition of the body and can be a hindrance to

losing weight; both because a person can store up to five pounds of waste and because the system is not healthy from toxic buildup. This produces a situation where the body senses it needs more nutrition, etc., which translates into more food.

When the system is toxic, you have less energy for exercise, which can lead to excess weight. In many cases of weight problems, there was toxicity of the colon. Parasites are another toxicity problem that can interfere with weight loss.
One of the first things that you can do when starting on your lifestyle change to eat better is to perform a colonic cleansing. If you have any colon problems, such as colitis or IBS, please check with your doctor first.

Colon cleansing can be tricky to do yourself. If you have any nervousness or misgivings about this, please consult a qualified natural health professional who administers colonics.

Parasites are often an obscure cause of colon toxicity, low energy, and weight imbalance. They are easier to pick up than you might think. Some sources include walking barefoot in the yard (and house, if you have indoor pets), eating lettuce or other leafy greens that have not been properly cleansed, swimming in creeks, eating improperly cooked meats, etc.

2. Liver.
The liver is such a vital, organ to the overall health of the

body. It's impossible for us to maintain any level of good health with an unhealthy liver. Due to high pollution levels in air, water and food, a liver cleanse at least 3-4 times a year is recommended. An effective liver cleanse can take weeks. Just taking something for a few days is not sufficient. Also, if you work in any environment where you are normally in contact with more than a fair share of pollution or toxicity—car mechanics, bus drivers, beauticians, painters, etc.—then you probably need to look at doing a liver cleanse even more often. If you haven't done a good liver cleanse within at least the past six months to a year, a toxic liver may be part of your inability to stay with a dietary program and lose weight. One of the best herbs for cleansing the liver is milk thistle.

3. Blood. If the colon and/or liver are toxic, the blood may also be toxic. Again, in support of the body system working to lose the extra weight, it is good to cleanse the blood. A very gentle and effective blood cleanse might include red clover tea and burdock root capsules. Try to do a blood cleanse at least once a year. Red Clover tea and Burdock Root are two of the better known blood cleansers. Red Clover is gentle and very effective, even for children. Burdock Root is more thorough so anyone with serious conditions would have to go slower on their detox with Burdock than with Red Clover.

4. Anti-Yeast Check. Rule out systemic yeast. This is another hidden and very insidious obstacle to weight loss. Make sure that you don't have Candida Albicans. If you do have it, there are ways to deal with it. Research and find a

good formula (caprylic acid will probably be in it when you find it) the South American herb Pau d'Arco is also excellent. Cut sugar out altogether. If you have systemic yeast, it is a must for you to stop use of sugar because sugar feeds the yeast.

The following questionnaire is from the book "The Yeast Connection", by William G. Crook, M.D.

SECTION A: HISTORY

1. Have you ever taken tetracyclines (Sumycin®, Panmycin®, Vibramycin®, Minocin®, etc.) or other antibiotics for acne for 1 month or longer?   35 points

2. Have you, at any time in your life, taken other "broad spectrum" antibiotics for respiratory, urinary or other infections (for 2 months or longer, or in shorter courses 4 or more times in a 1 year period?)   35 points
3. Have you taken a broad spectrum antibiotic drug, even a single course?   6 points

4. Have you, at any time in your life, been bothered by persistent prostatitis, vaginitis or other problems affecting your reproductive organs?   25 points

5. Have you been pregnant   2 or more times   5 points
                             1 time   3 points

6. Have you taken birth control pills for

more than 2 years?   15 points
For 6 months to 2 years?   8 points

7. Have you taken Prednisone, Decadron®, or other cortisone type drugs for

     more than 2 weeks   15 points
     2 weeks or less?   6 points

8. Does exposure to perfumes, insecticides, fabric shop odors and other chemicals provoke

     Moderate to severe symptoms 20
     Mild symptoms?   5

9. Are your symptoms worse on damp, muggy days or in moldy places?   20

10. Have you had athlete's foot, ringworm, "jock itch", or other chronic fungus infections of the skin or nails?

     Severe or persistent   20
     Mild to moderate   10

11. Do you crave sugar?   10
12. Do you crave breads?   10

13. Do you crave alcoholic beverages?   10

14. Does tobacco smoke *really* bother you?   10

    Total Score, Section A   ________

SECTION B: MAJOR SYMPTOMS

For each of your symptoms, enter the appropriate figure in the point score column:
If a symptom is *occasional or mild*....................score 3 points
If a symptom is *frequent and/or moderately severe*.....6 points
If a symptom is *severe and/or disabling*......................9 points

1. Fatigue or lethargy
2. Feeling of being "drained"
3. Depression
4. Poor memory
5. Feeling "spacey" or "unreal"
6. Inability to make decisions
7. Numbness, burning or tingling
8. Headache
9. Muscle aches
10. Muscle weakness or paralysis
11. Pain and/or swelling in joints
12. Abdominal pain
13. Constipation and/or diarrhea
14. Bloating, belching or intestinal gas
15. Troublesome vaginal burning, itching or discharge
16. Prostatitis
17. Impotence
18. Loss of sexual desire or feeling
19. Endometriosis or infertility
20.Cramps and/or other menstrual irregularities

21. Premenstrual tension
22. Attacks of anxiety or crying
23. Cold hands or feet and/or chilliness
24. Shaking or irritable when hungry

Total Score, Section B _________

SECTION C: OTHER SYMPTOMS
(While these symptoms commonly occur in people with
yeast-connected illness they are also found in other
individuals)
For each of your symptoms, enter the appropriate figure in
the point score column:
If a symptom is *occasional or mild*..................score 1 point
"   " *frequent and/or moderately severe* 2 points
"   " *severe and/or disabling*   3 points

1. Drowsiness
2. Irritability or jitteriness
3. Lack of coordination
4. Inability to concentrate
5. Mood swings
6. Insomnia
7. Dizziness/loss of balance
8. Pressure above ears...feeling of head swelling
9. Tendency to bruise easily
10. Chronic rashes or itching
11. Numbness, tingling
12. Indigestion or heartburn
13. Food sensitivity or intolerance
14. Mucus in stools

15. Rectal itching
16. Dry mouth or throat
17. Rash or blisters in mouth, canker sores
18. Bad breath
19. Foot, hair, or body odor not relieved by washing
20. Nasal congestion or post nasal drip
21. Nasal itching
22. Sore throat
23. Laryngitis, loss of voice
24. Cough or recurrent bronchitis
25. Pain or tightness in chest
26. Wheezing or shortness of breath
27. Urinary frequency or urgency
28. Burning on urination
29. Spots in front of eyes or erratic vision
30. Burning or tearing of eyes
31. Recurrent infections or fluid in ears
32. Ear pain or deafness

Total Score, Section C............................._________
Total Score, Section A............................._________
Total Score, Section B............................._________

GRAND TOTAL SCORE..............................._________

The Grand Total Score will help you and your physician decide if your health problems are yeast connected. Scores in women will run higher as 7 items in the questionnaire apply exclusively to women, while only 2 apply exclusively to men.

Yeast-connected health problems are almost certainly present in women *with scores over 180,* in men *with scores over 140.*

Yeast-connected health problems are probably present in women with scores *over 120,* men with scores *over 90.*

Yeast-connected health problems are possibly present in women with scores *over 60,* in men with scores *over 40.*

With scores of less than 60 in women and 40 in men, yeasts are less apt to cause health problems.

HOW TO TREAT A YEAST INFECTION

For more in-depth advice, please consult your doctor or the book, "The Yeast Connection" by Dr. William G. Crook. Here are some important tips.

It is critical to eliminate, at least temporarily, any and all foods and condiments that contribute, either directly or indirectly to the formation and growth of yeast. One of the best ways is to change your diet.

If you aren't willing to change your diet, you won't be able to conquer your candida. So, for at least one week, change over to the following guidelines:

1. Your diet should include lots of nutritious food from a wide variety of sources.

2. You must avoid junk foods, foods which are overly processed, refined, and full of sugar, salt, food colorings, additives and hydrogenated vegetable oils.

3. Especially avoid all sugars, honey, molasses, etc. Sugar feeds candida just as fuel feeds a fire.

4. During the first week of your diet, focus on low carbohydrate vegetables, seafood, lean meats and eggs. You can also include a single portion of a whole grain at each meal.

5. Avoid all yeast containing foods. At the end of a week, if you've begun to feel better and your symptoms are calming down, challenge with yeast and see if it bothers you.

THE YEAST CHALLENGE

On the 8th day of your diet, break off a crumb of a brewer's yeast tablet and eat it. If you show no reaction in 10 minutes, eat a bigger crumb. Continue to eat additional pieces of the yeast tablet during the next hour. If you show no reaction to the first tablet, eat a second tablet several hours later. The next day eat a mushroom and try yeasty foods such as moldy-type cheese.

If these yeast challenges do not provoke symptoms, chances are you aren't allergic to yeast-containing foods and can consume them in moderation. This will make following the diet a lot easier for you.

However, don't go overboard and stuff yourself with yeasty foods everyday as you may develop an allergy to these foods (the more you eat of any food, especially if you eat it every day, the greater your chances of developing an allergy to the food).

Of course, if you develop symptoms while you're experimenting with yeast, stop. Don't make yourself sick. If you are uncertain or your symptoms are minor, wait two days and repeat the challenges.

6. If you pass the yeast challenge, rotate nuts and seeds into your diet. Also, add sprouts.

7. Avoid all fruits during the first three weeks of your diet. Although fruits are complex carbohydrates and furnish many excellent nutrients, they are easily converted into simple sugars in the intestinal tract. On the 21st day of your diet, do a fruit challenge.
      Take a small bite of banana. Ten minutes later, eat a second bite. If no reaction develops in the next hour, eat the whole banana. If you tolerate the banana without having symptoms, try strawberries, pineapple, or apple the next day. If you show no adverse reaction to these fruit challenges, most likely you can take fruit in moderation. But feel your way along and do not overdo it.
8. Rotate your diet so as to get foods from a broad variety of sources. Also, rotating your diet may enable you to more

easily identify a food that may be disagreeing with you and causing symptoms.

FOODS YOU MUST AVOID

Sugar and Sugar-containing Foods: Sugar and other quick-acting carbohydrates, including sucrose, fructose, maltose, lactose, glycogen, glucose, mannitol, sorbitol, galactose, monosaccharides andpolysachharides. Also avoid honey, molasses, maple syrup, maple sugar, date sugar and turbinado sugar.

Packaged and Processed Foods: Canned, bottled, boxed and other packaged and processed foods usually contain hidden ingredients and refined sugar products.

You'll not only need to avoid these sugar-containing foods the early weeks of your diet, *you'll need to avoid them indefinitely.*

Avoid yeasty foods the first 7-10 days of your diet. Then do the yeast challenge as described later on. If you're allergic to yeast you'll need to continue to avoid yeast and mold-containing foods indefinitely. But if you aren't allergic to yeast, you can rotate yeast-containing foods into your diet and eat them in moderation.

Breads, Pastries and other raised bread products

Cheese: all cheeses including cheese products such as

Velveeta and other cheese containing snacks. Also avoid buttermilk, sour cream and sour milk products.

Alcoholic Beverages: including beer, vodka, rum, whiskey and other fermented liquors. Also cider and root beer.

Condiments, Sauces and Vinegar-containing foods: Mustard, ketchup, Worcestershire, Accent, (monosodium glutamate—MSG), steak, barbecue, soy and shrimp sauces, pickles, pickled vegetables, sauerkraut, green olives, horseradish, mince meat and tamari. Vinegar and all kinds of vinegar-containing foods such as mayonnaise and salad dressing. (Freshly squeezed lemon juice may be used as a substitute for vinegar and salad dressings).

Malt Products: Malted milk drinks, cereals and candy. (Malt is sprouted grain that is kiln-dried and used in the preparation of many processed foods and beverages).

Processed and Smoked Meats: Pickled and smoked meats including sausages, hot dogs, corned beef, pastrami, and pickled tongue.

Edible Fungi: All types of mushrooms, morels, and truffles.

Melons: Watermelon, honeydew melon and especially cantaloupe. (Careful washing of melons before cutting may enable melons to be tolerated.)

Coffee and Tea

Fruit Juices: Either canned, bottled or frozen. Exception: freshly prepared juice.

Dried & Candied Fruits: Raisins, apricots, dates, prunes, etc.

Leftovers: Molds grow in leftover food unless it's properly refrigerated. Freezing is better.

FOODS TO EAT CAUTIOUSLY

High Carbohydrate Vegetables
Sweet Corn, Lima Beans, English Peas, White Potatoes (baked), Winter Squash, Acorn, or Butternut, Sweet Potatoes, Beans and Peas

Whole Grains
Barley, Corn, Millet, Oats, Rice, Wheat

Breads, Biscuits & Muffins
All breads, biscuits, and muffins should be made with baking powder or baking soda as a leavening agent. DO NOT use yeast unless you pass the yeast challenge. To avoid yeast and to obtain more vitamins and minerals, use whole wheat flour or stone ground cornmeal.

FOODS YOU CAN EAT FREELY

Vegetables
Most of these vegetables contain lots of fiber and are relatively low in carbohydrates. They can be fresh or

frozen, eaten cooked or raw.
Asparagus, Beets, Broccoli, Brussel Sprouts, Cabbage,
Carrots, Cauliflower, Celery, Cucumbers, Eggplant, Green
Pepper, Greens (Spinach, Mustard, Beet, Collards, Kale),
Lettuce (all varieties), Okra, Onions, Parsley, Radishes,
Soybeans, String Beans, Tomatoes (fresh), Turnips

Meats and Eggs
Chicken, Turkey, Salmon, Mackerel, Cod, Sardines, Tuna,
Other fresh or frozen fish that isn't breaded, Shrimp,
Lobster, Crab, and other seafood, Beef (lean cuts),
Pork(lean cuts), Lamb, Wild Game, Eggs. (these are just
suggestions! Of course eat only the types you like)

Nuts, Seeds & Oils (unprocessed)
Note: nuts may disagree with you and cause symptoms,
especially if you're allergic to yeasts and molds.
Almonds, Brazil Nuts, Cashews, Filberts, Pecans, Pumpkin
Seeds, Oils: Linseed Safflower, Sunflower, Soy, Walnut,
Corn. Butter.

To Drink
Water

When you follow these dietary recommendations, you
should improve. The first two or three days will be the most
difficult, but please persevere, it will be worth it. You may
even be able to "cheat" now and then without causing
problems. But if you aren't careful and overindulge in junk
foods and sweets, your health problems will usually return.

Yeast problems may also be helped through Homeopathy.
To learn more about this, consult a qualified practitioner.

Keeping Candida under control requires more than
medication and a special diet. To go into this in the detail
necessary to do it justice would require another book.

Other ways to cleanse the body system:

For reducing heavy metal toxins, the herb Cilantro is good.
Just munch on it fresh or use it in cooking or as a tea.

Other cleansing herbal teas: dandelion root, burdock root,
milk thistle. If you are pregnant or nursing, check with a
professional before using any herbs.

Eat washed fresh fruits and vegetables. Try to get organic if
at all possible.

Consider food allergies as culprits. As with the candida
diet, eliminate possible allergens for at least 3 weeks.
Common allergy-inducing foods are: Wheat, Corn, Eggs,
and Milk and Soy products. If you feel better (more energy,
clearing of nasal passages, weight loss, etc.) then you know
what not to eat. Remember to drop only one food at a time
or you won't know what it is you're allergic to!

These little ingredients cause big problems with weight loss
and good health in general. Please consider giving up:

   *Refined Sugar

*Grains
*MSG
*Aspartame, Splenda and other chemical sweeteners

There are healthy alternatives to sugar, but you must develop a taste for them. Stevia is the best. Find out the other names MSG goes by, added to foods in a hidden way.

OMEGA THREE FATS ARE ESSENTIAL TO YOUR HEALTH. You can get them from cod liver oil, Omega3 fish oil or flaxseed.

Unfortunately nearly all fish are contaminated with mercury and should ideally be avoided. You will want to identify a clean source of fish oil. If you are vegetarian, you can use flaxseed instead. Make sure you use FRESH flaxseeds or the oil and keep them refrigerated.

If you are outside in the summer a lot then you should not take cod liver oil as you will run the risk of overdosing on vitamin D, which is produced by the body when exposed to sunlight.

You should then take fish oil capsules. The standard fish oil capsule is 180 mg of EPA and 120 mg of DHA. You should take about one capsule for every ten pounds of body weight, ideally in two divided doses. So if you weigh 160 pounds you would take 8 capsules twice a day. If you have problems with burping them up, you will want to think about taking them on an empty stomach.

You can tell if a fish oil capsule is fresh by puncturing it
and seeing if there is any "fishy" aftertaste. This is usually a
sign of rancid fat and a sign of an inferior product.

Consult a trusted naturopathic doctor for more advice,
testing for vitamin D levels, and how best to supplement
for deficiencies. Some allopathic doctors will test for
vitamin D, as this has become more popular.

When you take fish oil supplements or cod liver oil please
be sure and take one vitamin E 400 unit supplement per day
as this will help serve to protect the fat from oxidation.
This is less of a problem with the cod liver oil as the
vitamin D by itself is a very powerful anti-oxidant. In cold
and flu season, a six-foot 200 pound person can take as
much as 12000 IU of vitamin D a day to lessen a cold/flu,
up to 6000 or 8000 as a preventative. Adjust dosage for
your height and weight, or consult a nutritional doctor.

You will also need extra amounts of the often forgotten oil
soluble vitamin, vitamin K. If you are juicing plenty of
green vegetables and taking the cod liver oil or fish oil with
the juice you should absorb the vitamin K in the vegetable
juice. But, if you have osteoporosis or osteopenia, you will
want to add an extra 1000 mcg (1 mg of vitamin K per day.

Typically our diet contains far too much omega 6 fats.
Authorities looking at the dietary ratio of omega 6 to
omega3 fatty acids suggest that in early human history the
ratio was about 1:1. Today most Americans eat a dietary
ratio that falls between 20:1 and 50:1. The optimal ratio is

most likely closer to the original ratio of 1:1. For most of us this means greatly reducing the omega-6 fatty acids we consume and increasing the amount of omega-3 fatty acids.

We get ALL the omega 6 and omega 9 fat we need from food and cooking (olive oil is wonderful and healthy to cook with). We do NOT need to take any supplements for these fats.

It is highly recommended to avoid sunflower, corn, soy, safflower, canola, or products that contain these oils. That is, no hydrogenated or partially hydrogenated fats, no margarine, no vegetable oil, no shortening. These oils are full of omega 6 fats and will only make your omega 6 to omega 3 ratio worse. Not to mention that these oils are processed in a way that is destructive to our body's system, (trans-fats) and they are genetically modified.

Acceptable oils will be a high quality extra virgin olive oil, coconut oil, avocados, and organic butter, or better yet grass-fed organic butter.

Another way to improve your omega 6:3 ratio is to change the type of meat you are eating. You could eat more game meat like venison, or other game animals that are raised only on grass type foods. However, these are hard to find and generally more expensive than beef. Buffalo meat is another good choice. Since nearly all cattle are grain fed before slaughter, if you eat most traditionally raised beef, it will usually worsen you omega 6 to omega 3 ratio. Normally a good ratio for omega 6:3 in fish is 2 or 3 to 1, the lower the better. Grass fed beef can be higher in Omega 3 than fish, with a 6 to 3 ratio of 0.16 to 1.

To get the necessary Omega-3 fatty acids, you should consider eating meat that is allowed to "free-range", or in the case of cattle, to be grass-fed. Unfortunately, you cannot buy this grass-fed beef at your local grocery store. Check into individual farmers and your health food store, or go online.

You need to be careful as many stores will advertise grass-fed beef but it really isn't. They do this because ALL cattle are grass fed, but the key is what they are fed the months before being processed. Most all cattle are shipped to giant feed lots and fed corn to fatten them up. You will need to call the person who actually grew the beef, NOT the store manager, to find out the truth.

Step C. BUILD THE BODY SYSTEM

Of course, you've made tremendous progress with tapping
away your food addictions. You might not think you need
to do anything else. For some people, this may be true. For
others, you might want to help your body even more by
supporting your new-found health through eating good
food, using good fats, supplements and exercise.

Now that you've gotten your body cleansed and feeling
healthier, you can turn your attention to building your body
system up. This is a critical step on the path to "permanent"
weight loss. The goal is for you to lose what you want to
lose, for good.

As always, if you have any serious medical condition or are
under the doctor's care, please check with your doctor
before adding these or any other healthcare products to your
regimen

ENZYMES AND WEIGHT LOSS:

One of the essential keys to weight-loss may be the action
of enzymes. Lipase for example is found abundantly in raw
foods but few of us eat enough raw foods to get enough
lipase to burn even a normal amount of fat, let alone any
excess. Lipase is a fat splitting enzyme that helps the body
in digestion, fat distribution and the burning of fat for
energy. Lipase activity breaks down and dissolves fat
around the body. Without lipase, fat stagnates and
accumulates in organs, arteries and capillaries. You will

also notice it on hips, thighs, buttocks and the stomach.

Protease is another crucial enzyme for maintaining a healthy body. The two main roles that Protease plays are to break down proteins and eliminate toxins. The elimination of toxins is crucial for anyone who is burning fat. Your body stores excess toxins in your body fat. As your body begins to burn this fat the toxins are released back into your system. This can sometimes cause water retention, flu-like symptoms, tiredness and bloating. Since Protease attacks and eliminates toxins, it is important to have extra protease during fat loss. Ask your local health food store or healthcare professional for good supplements.

STEP D: FIND THE RIGHT PROGRAM FOR YOU

The best diet programs will advocate a healthy balance of good foods, moderate exercise and nutritional supplementation. Use what works for you but do the work you need to do before you start, to insure permanent weight loss in a health way.

Of course, no weight loss program would be complete without including exercise. The important thing with exercise is

    A. to pick something you enjoy doing –Brisk walks, preferably outside, dancing, swimming, etc.
    B. something that isn't complicated, doesn't involve

a lot of equipment, etc.

Remember, you can always do EFT to overcome any mental obstacles that prevent you from exercising.

If you cleanse the body, support it with the right enzymes, vitamins and minerals, and food and work daily to reduce your stress level, these will be helpful along with EFT to balance your body and achieve health and weight loss.

FINALLY....
There are many good books out there that go into more depth than I can here concerning particular areas of natural health, nutrition, supplements, food, longevity, stress reduction, and eating well. I have included an extensive bibliography of books that I highly recommend, based on over 25 years of experience in the alternative health care field. This is not to say you need to do *all* of these things, pick and choose, do a little at a time. DO what feels best for *you*.

Remember: you are a beautiful person!

All the best to you in your achievement of health, happiness, and balance!

BIBLIOGRAPY

The Plan, Lyn-Genet Recitas
Raise Your Vibration, Nogah Lord
Today's Herbal Health, Louise Tenney
Fit For Life I and II, Harvey and Marilyn Diamond
The Yeast Connection, William G. Crook, M.D.
The Complete Book of Chinese Health and Healing, Daniel
Reid
The Tao of Health, Sex, and Longevity, Daniel Reid
Natural Health, Natural Medicine, Andrew Weil, M.D.
Lick the Sugar Habit, Nancy Appleton, Ph.D.
Prescription for Nutritional Healing, Balch
In Bad Taste: The MSG Symptom Complex, by George R.
Schwartz and Kathleen A. Schwartz.
Get Healthy Now, Gary Null

There are many more excellent books out there. Look at
your local library or online. Trust sources that have been
around for at least a few years.

Remember: *You are a beautiful person!*
             You can do it!

I wish you all the best in your achievements!

ABOUT THE AUTHOR

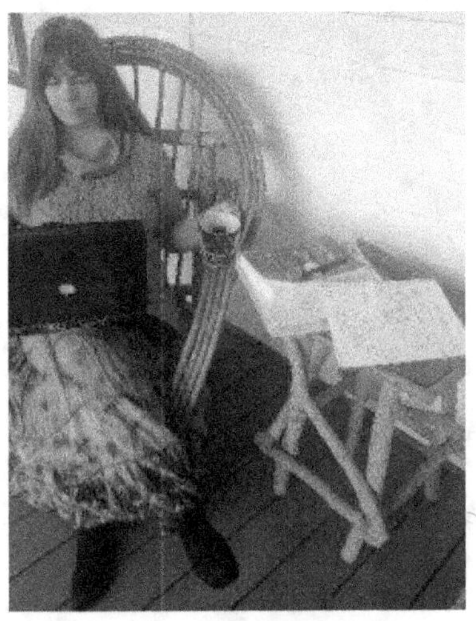

Janet Brown has been a Master Herbalist since 1987 and written over one hundred documents on herbal and natural healing. An EFT practitioner since 2001, she has a success rate with her clients of over 95%. She teaches EFT classes and workshops and has written two books on using EFT. She has also written over 100 workshops and mini-books since 1987, when she began studying herbs and other natural healing methods.

She has received a B.A. in English Literature from Michigan State University, and herbal training from Michigan State University, and Clayton School of Natural Health.